Swift Meditation

Power to Everyone

Aegis CIPL

Table of Contents

Introduction

Meditation is a process that has existed since the beginning of humanity. Homo sapiens have used it in some form, knowingly or unknowingly. If there is a mind with conscious control, the process of meditation can exist. It is interesting to note that the conscious mind causes most of our actions and decisions, but it can also leave it messy with over-thinking and negative thoughts. Animals have brains but they are behind in evolution. Their reasoning, analytical and creative thinking process is either nil or far behind humans. They cannot think logically with limited ability to identify patterns. They can neither create knowledge nor can transfer their experience or understanding to others. They can communicate only with limited sounds and actions. Their memories and sense of time are limited. Animals act based on superior instincts (to humans), which help them survive their dangerous environment. The whole purpose of animal life is existence and procreation. As their mind is not complex and focused on tasks necessary for existence, they do not need meditation for focus and clarity. But the human brain is mysteriously different. Its power has allowed us to rule planet Earth and claim the right of ownership on other planets.

The human brain is one of the most interesting and evolved bio-organ present in our universe. It is still a mystery for scientists and spiritual masters. Present technology has only partially understood the human brain. Doctors and researchers agree that a lot more is yet to be explored. A human brain is an exciting place, full of action. The small physical mass consists of uncountable elements which make every human unique and different from another. The interactions between these elements develop a unique personality. The emotions, thoughts, experiences, motivations and perceptions make a human a person with a personality. The mind with consciousness differs from the brain.

The Mind of the Brain

The brain is a complex physical organ that is the central processing unit, controlling the whole body and its functions. It operates with electrical pulses and the release of chemicals to control certain activities. A body without a brain is not alive, it cannot function. But the mind resides in the brain in consciousness, intelligence, thoughts, emotions, perception, imagination, judgment, memory and knowledge. The mind allows a person to visualize and think logically. This is a place where creativity, rational thinking, values, beliefs and behavior resides. It gives a person her personality and character. The mind of a person exists only in nonphysical form. The brain of almost every human is similar but the mind is different. The mind is a choice that can be developed and enhanced but the brain takes birth with the body and dies with it.

The analogy that the brain is the hardware and the mind is software is flawed. The mind can transform the person and even change the brain. It can perform tasks not yet been understood by science. It can self-heal and can cure the disturbed mind of others. It can connect and develop the virgin minds to open infinite possibilities. Meditation is the key to unlock several mysteries of the brain.

Mind's Segments

The mind can be segmented into three parts, conscience, subconscious and unconscious. The conscious mind is concerned about the awareness of the present. It allows us to think rationally or creatively about the actions to be taken. The physical actions are also controlled by the conscious mind, for example, driving a car, writing an article, climbing up the stairs or presenting at a conference. The conscious mind is supported by the massive storage in the subconscious mind, where all our memories, experiences, beliefs, values and information is stored. The subconscious mind can be considered several times bigger than the conscious mind and is responsible for the personality, character and attitude of an individual. The conscious mind is always backed by the subconscious mind for its operations and actions. For example, the automatic functions while driving the car are stored in the subconscious mind. The unconscious mind manages the functioning of all activities of the body and mind which cannot be controlled consciously. For example, the beating of the heart, managing information between the mind and the body and balancing the chemicals present in different organs. All three minds work in coordination with the common objective to make you a healthy human, allowing you to achieve your goals while being happy.

Meditation is controlling and expanding the mind, which is beneficial in every possible way. Meditation is considered mysterious, complex and time-consuming as it is marketed as the science of the mind and body. The objective of this book is to make the whole process simple to achieve most of its benefits in the least possible time. The solution is Swift Meditation.

The Objective of this Book

Meditation has been the buzzword of print and online media for the last few decades. Check any media channel and loads of content about meditation can be found in it. The massive number of books and the amount of published content are enough to intimidate any normal person with the concept of meditation. It seems so complex and out of reach. Years of practice and guidance of spiritual gurus are necessary to reap the benefits of meditation. It is the reason that most people do not understand the concept of meditation, even if they fascinate it.

It is also assumed that integrating meditation in daily life would require a certain time commitment from our busy schedule. As most of humanity is already short of time due to their hectic working hours and personal commitments, meditation takes the back seat. It is generally postponed to the later years of age.

It must be understood that meditation is natural to every human. It is the need of the mind and brain to help it function most productively. It can be used by anyone, anywhere and in any condition. Even professionals with a deficiency of time can use meditation to enhance the quality of their lives.

This book will solve the mystery around the concept of meditation. Instead of comprehending hundreds of pages of information, the fundamental concept of meditation can be explained in few sentences. Once the basic concepts are clear, meditation can be experienced through simple techniques. The benefits associated with deep relaxation will be enough to stimulate any person to explore further. The understanding and practice of Swift Meditation is the beginning of integrating meditation in life.

The main focus of this book is to introduce the concept of Swift Meditation (called SM in short). The meaning of Swift Meditation is to get into a meditative state in the least possible time, using unique and effective techniques. This book will describe the concept and the techniques.

One objective of the book is to keep it short and easy to understand. The language used is simple for any person to easily understand the concepts described in the book. We understand the time limitations of the people and the challenge to complete a whole book to grasp the fundamental idea.

This book will also discuss several techniques which can be used for Swift Meditation. Any practitioner can use one or more of these techniques to get into the meditative state for relaxation and control. This will be the first step in the journey towards deeper meditation.

The Concept

Meditation is the process to put the mind in a deeply relaxed state. This is when the mind is free of any stress, tension, negative thoughts, fear or anxiety. If the brain is considered a machine operating at high capacity, it would need regular relaxation to improve performance. Sleeping is one way to relax the mind, but any deeper relaxed state would always be welcomed. Meditation allows any person to reach that deeper relaxation state.

The mind is an active organ of the human body. It is constantly working unconsciously and subconsciously. An awake person is using her conscious mind for actions and thought process in the present moment. The thoughts in the mind can be generated either consciously or subconsciously. Even though the attention is given to only a few thoughts every day, the unattended thoughts suck the energy out of the brain. They add to the existing stress of the brain. These irrelevant thoughts add nil value and serve no purpose. Most thoughts are generated through information captured by our five senses. A happy and controlled person would minimize the flow of thoughts in her mind to enjoy complete freedom from tiring stream of information and needless processing which wastes precious energy.

We will aim to gain that control over the stream of thoughts.

The source of noise and irrelevant thoughts

Our mind is always busy capturing, processing and interpreting information received from various sources. Before we understand the process to free our mind from thoughts to achieve Swift Meditation, we must understand the different sources producing thoughts in mind.

1. **Human Senses**- The five senses of Sight, Sound, Smell, Taste, and Touch. These senses are always working hard to capture the information from the environment and the world.

2. **Subconscious mind**- Most of our memories, feelings and experiences are stored in the

subconscious mind. This active storage is always ready to pop up information at the stimulus provided by the conscious mind. And, our active brain is good at producing a constant stream of the stimulus.

3. **Emotions**- are the fundamental reason for human action. Some of our strong emotions are love, anger, compassion and hate. Most of our actions are dictated by our emotions as they drive every human. Emotions, both good and bad, generate steady torrents of thoughts.

4. **External influences**- The attention-grabbing events of the environment also capture attention to generate unsolicited thoughts.

5. **Thoughts**- Even existing thoughts are generating connected thoughts like a tree structure. These trees are constantly growing to become big, dense and complex.

6. **Data processing**- The mind is always capturing and clenching data to produce information, allowing us to take decisions and actions. Mind rarely differentiates between relevant and irrelevant information, it absorbs all. It rejects irrelevant information during processing, but it is time-consuming and wastes precious energy. This processing can be minimized by reducing the number of captured data by the mind

and automatic differentiation between relevant and irrelevant information.

The problem with unattended thoughts

Most thoughts existing in the mind are unattended thoughts. This is similar to noise in the mind, interfering with every task mind is struggling to perform. The majority of the mind's clutter is not generated consciously, instead, physical senses and information from the subconscious mind keep the mind engaged by forcing unsolicited analysis. For example, a pungent smell can raise several thoughts in the mind, like:

- What type of smell is it?
- From where is it coming?
- Where have I smelt it before?
- The source of the smell?
- How long will it remain?
- Is it related to me in any way?
- Is it dangerous?
- Should I ignore it?
- Who is responsible for it?

- Why should this be my course of action?
- What should I do now?

The mind inherently raises questions while automatically trying to answer them. The whole process is fast, lasting few seconds but it consumes precious energy, tiring the mind. The presence of a large number of thoughts in the mind does not mean that the mind could make the sense of them all, instead, it uses tags to differentiate between them. These tags can later create connections with the existing information present in the mind. If thought is interesting, then it can be explored further, otherwise, it remains an unattended thought. It depends upon the priority attached to a specific thought. As we have limited energy and time only a few thoughts can be attended at a point in time. This means that most thoughts will remain unattended, allowing them to put stress on the mind. The unattended thoughts drain the energy of the body. Usable energy present in the mind is proportional to the ability to minimize the number of irrelevant thoughts in the mind.

Meditation drives out all the unreasonable or illogical thoughts from the mind to save energy to perform reasonable and important actions. The best way would be to block the entry of junk information to the mind, even if physical senses capture it from the environment. This process cannot be repeated consciously, instead, it must be automatic. The successful application of this principle would allow a concentration on important thoughts and ideas to extract value. It is not simple as the majority of humanity cannot meditate successfully. Few people who have the command over their mind through meditation can have control over their emotions, thoughts and thought processes.

Swift Meditation can help in limiting the flow of vague thoughts while driving out most of the unreasonable thoughts from the mind. Regular practice would improve the command over the process to make it automatic.

Birth of Stress

Mental Stress is the major reason for diseases and low productivity. A large number of unattended thoughts struggling for attention contribute to stress. This could be due to pressure at work, heavy responsibility, lack of control, uncertainty, tough challenges or anything else which increases the rate of thoughts generation in mind.

Unattended thoughts are just one reason for the stress, there could be several other reasons responsible for stressing the mind. Let's look at some of the reasons.

The Reasons for Stress

- The number of thoughts coming to the mind can be large. If you cannot manage the number of thoughts by having control over your mind, then it would lead to stress. Few people have those abilities who have attained it through focus and meditation. Swift Meditation can also help in managing the number of thoughts in the mind.

- The ability to think is unique to humans but it may lead to side effects of over-thinking, which is unnecessarily thinking about something. Over-thinking is a habit and a choice that can be corrected consciously. In most cases over-thinking never leads to any positive result. A person may think too much about something, which is not even real. For example, a person may think about an event not yet happened or have no possibility of happening. An individual can think negatively about something bad in her life, getting trapped in it. The habit of over-thinking is never helpful, instead, it is one reason for anxiety, a major generator of irrelevant thoughts.

- Fear is natural to every person. It is a way for the mind to show discomfort about something or someone. It can be real or fictitious as the mind is good at making stories. Usually, fear exists only in the mind without any reality. A person afraid of ghosts can find the presence of evil anywhere or in every person. This fear is self-generated and can be solved only by the conscious efforts of the person. If fear is not controlled (or managed) consciously, it will become overpowering, disrupting the natural course of life. Fear is also one of the reasons people get stressed about something imaginary.

- Confusion is another reason for stress. A person can be confused about taking a decision or a course of action. There could be various other reasons for the confusion, lack of self-belief, lack of information, distrust or fear. It depends upon the right actions taken by an individual to manage the state of confusion. A person learning to get clarity in mind will be more productive and better at taking action. The ability to control thoughts through mental clarity can reduce the intensity of confusion.

- Humans are made up of emotions, lots of colorful emotions. They are both the source of fear, pain, happiness and fun. Emotions can make us weak but also act as a source of strength. Human decisions and most actions are the product of emotions. A complex mix of feelings can also lead to frequent irrational decisions, even after prolonged suffering. Emotions cannot be segregated into good or bad, instead, the perception and the actions based upon a specific emotion defines it, giving it meaning. For example, anger can allow a person to use its energy for achieving something great, or infatuation (disguised as love) can force a person to take wrong actions. Emotions not adding value to a person's life can be the source of stress, which are necessary to be managed.

- Expectations are the source of conflicts and anguish. Expectations can be from the self or others. Most relationships are based on expectations which can be personal or professional. For example, two romantic partners can expect trust and respect from each other, while business partners can expect transparency and mutual benefits. If expectations are not met, it leads to stress, pain and a burst of negative emotions. Some saints have declared that expectations are the root cause of all the problems, 'so stop expecting anything from anyone,' which is impractical. If you live in a society with a social life, you will have expectations. The best way is to be rational by having reasonable expectations from people and yourself. We must have control over our emotions so that if expectations are not met, it only becomes a lesson, not a bad action.

- Even physical strain leads to stress. A person working hard on a factory shop floor can be stressed due to physical fatigue. Proper diet and physical fitness can help in managing physical strain. A person should also be aware of the limits of his body for physical strain.

- Then there could be various other reasons for stress unique for a person and her environment.

The Power of Meditation

Since the beginning of thinking intelligently, humans have been searching to understand the mystery of the mind. They used it in different conditions and environments to examine its effectiveness. It was discovered that a peaceful and clear mind can be the key to creativity and logical thoughts. As life and human lifestyle became complex, so the reasons to disturb the mind. Different human senses, instead of helping the mind, became the source of noise and vague data. As human senses are extremely sensitive, they capture each and everything around them. The noise produced by our scooter, the heated communication between two friends, the change of temperature due to air conditioners, the strong smell of perfume and the sharp colors used in a banner advertisement. Everything is a source of some data picked up by the senses and pushed to the mind. It is left our brain to process that information and segregate based on priority. This is a big task as the flow of information is never-ending. This heavy work tires the brain.

If a process could automatically segregate the information from the noise, rejecting it, the brain would be less stressed allowing it to focus on other relevant areas. The selected information is segregated based upon relevance and priority. This is an appropriate and much productive way to manage information. Meditation helps in keeping the brain healthy and mind efficient and effective. It does not allow the mind to be overburdened by vague thoughts, allowing clarity.

Meditation is not only good for the brain and mind but the whole body benefits with regular practice. It keeps the brain relaxed and the mind efficient. It manages stress to ensure effective usage of our precious energy. The functioning of the body is directly related to the mind. A sound mind exists in a healthy body and vice versa. It has been scientifically proven that regular practice of meditation results in happiness, clarity and prosperity.

Meditation is not commonly used

The benefits of meditation are known for centuries and millenniums, but only a small percentage of people use it. Most of the people in the present time are aware of this word and many people have desired to experience its power, but only a few took the next step in practicing meditation. The reasons could be:

- <u>Right Information</u>: Lack of effective information required for the practice of meditation. Even with a massive amount of information available in the form of books, articles, videos and audios, people aren't able to find the required information in a simple format.

- <u>Lack of motivation</u>: As only a few people feel the intense need for meditation, due to their extraordinary situations. Time is considered the most precious resource in the present century and every day many pending issues are in the queue, waiting for attention.

- <u>Mysterious</u>: Mystery associated with the practice of meditation also acts as a deterrent. It is considered an ancient practice used by saints, angels and Gods. For some people, it seems distant and disconnected. Though in the present time, many practitioners and professionals have brought meditation to the mass media.

- <u>Time</u>: Many people have a limitation of time due to their busy schedules and constant deadlines. They are not ready to invest time to understand the concept and gain enough expertise to experience value from meditation. This reason becomes one of the top excuses for procrastination.

- <u>Bad Elements</u>: As meditation is becoming popular many wrong people have entered the field who have little or no knowledge about meditation. They are present only to extract money from other people. This bad experience also desists people for new experimentation.

- <u>Patience</u>: Some people do not have enough patience to experience the power of meditation. Focus and the control of the mind do not come easy, it requires dedicated practice for a long time to experience its value. The casual practice of some people does not allow them to see any value in meditation.

- <u>Unfashionable</u>: Meditation being an ancient practice sometimes may look uncool. The present generation may not want to get associated with something which they cannot share on social media. Meditation is not about being visible to others, a selfie in the meditative state cannot be taken. Some people may not find value in something which cannot be shared on

Instagram. The mentality is now slowly changing as many celebrities, professionals and other people are understanding the benefits of meditation.

These are some of the specified reasons but people can have their unique excuses for postponing the practice of meditation. Swift Meditation can solve this problem.

Precautions in Meditation

Meditation is a powerful process to enhance the abilities of the mind and body to use it effectively and efficiently. It energizes the body and brings clarity to the thinking process. There are various ways to experience meditation and go deeper into it. Some people chant mantras while others use the process of visualization to get into meditation. Silent observation is also a way to experience deeper meditation, for example, observing and experiencing the way of breathing or activities of a specific part of the body or just observing nature.

Meditation is an efficacious way to calm the mind and to have better control over emotions. Whatever be the type of meditation the objective remains the same. It is the natural way of the mind to concentrate by driving out thoughts, making it clean and fresh. Meditation allows the mind to reenergize to work effectively and efficiently.

The objective of meditation should not be to detach from reality, by using visualization to live in a virtual world. People scared of pain or fear could use this enlightening process to immune themselves from emotions, in the hope to avoid any suffering, which is an inherent part of being human and is essential to make us better by constant improvements.

Swift Meditation

The objective of Swift Meditation is to make a person experience meditation instantly, in the simplest possible way. Swift Meditation may not be as deep as the main meditation but it is relaxing and can help in extracting the main benefits of meditation. This can be the start of the process of meditation and understanding its power. Swift Meditation solves most of the problems associated with meditation and answers unanswered questions. People cannot find the reasons to ignore it or to procrastinate. The choice of experiencing meditation can be in an instant. Swift Meditation can be as easy as posting an update on social media.

We should Discuss Swift Meditation

A question may arise that if the meditation exists then what is the need for Swift Meditation. A part of the answer has been discussed in the previous sections of the book.

Meditation seems complex and intimidating for most people. The lack of time and resources resists the need to gain value from meditation. Swift Meditation solves these problems allowing every person interested in meditation to experience the focus, clarity and relaxation experienced in the process of meditation. This can be attained with Swift Meditation in few minutes, even if the person is a beginner in the field of meditation.

- The process of Swift Meditation is not religious. It is not related to any specific religion or spiritual thought. It is a simple and effective technique for relaxation and focus.

- Swift Meditation can be achieved in few minutes of practice. This has no time constraints and can be used by any individual regardless of any differences.

- The concept associated with Swift Meditation is simple and can be understood easily by anyone irrespective of the educational background. An illiterate person can experience a similar level of mental balance just like a person with professional degrees, initiated by Swift Meditation.

- It is not mysterious, instead, it is a simple technique to relax the mind and gain focus for the task in hand. The concept of Swift Meditation is based on the ancient practice but is much simpler and modern, considering the limitations and requirements of the present time.

- It can be used for any work or profession. A worker on the road can use it effectively just the way any lawyer, consultant or politician.

- The proper use of Swift Meditation can raise the overall productivity of a person or a team, which will be visible in results and output.

- Swift Meditation can add value to life and work in various ways. It can enhance the personal life of the person practicing it and can improve the quality and productivity of professional work.

The Need – Lack of Time

The process of meditation is complex and mysterious,

generally inaccessible to most people. Swift Meditation can be accessed by interested people who want to get the benefits of deep relaxation. This is a simple way to meditate that can be learned immediately and started with few hours of practice.

Meditation is always considered good for mental and physical health due to its positive effects on the mind and body. Meditation is beneficial in numerous diseases either by curing it or alleviating the intensity of the symptoms. It is an integral part of the ancient practice of yoga. Meditation has been used for thousands of years in various regions in different forms such as religious practices or exercises for mental or physical wellbeing.

People are always short of time. They need an effective way to get the benefits of meditation without committing to long daily practice for years. Swift Meditation will open up a simple path to meditation without heavy commitments. It will allow them to meditate anytime, anywhere with no complex ritual.

The main cause of stress is the lack of mental and physical relaxation. Swift Meditation is focused on achieving the state of deep relaxation immediately. As this form of meditation can be performed anywhere without fanfare, it can provide constant dosages of deep relaxation anytime.

Swift Meditation is helpful

- Swift Meditation can be helpful for people new to meditation and also for seasoned practitioners. It is simple enough for people to start experiencing Swift Meditation immediately without long or hard practice. For experts in meditation, the process gives them a new tool to get into the state of meditation in few minutes.

- The objective of Swift Meditation is to open the doors of meditation for every interested individual. People may have different constraints, but the simplicity of Swift Meditation will allow meditation practice even in complex situations and conditions.

- This is especially beneficial for busy people who do not have time for their mental health. Swift Meditation can be the start of the actions to care for the mind and body. The performance and motivation of a healthy person will always be better. The enlightening experience of meditation will allow an individual to focus on other important areas of life including health and family. Swift Meditation will provide the constant dosages of mental relaxation which will be tremendously helpful for mental health.

- Meditation when integrated with yoga can be beneficial in several medical conditions and diseases. The focus on breathing, the calmness of mind, and the right stretching of muscles can bring wonders to human health. It can also open the locked doors of the mind to offer new solutions and ideas for the problems in hand.

- Meditation can improve the quality of decisions by bringing clarity and focus. The enhanced attention to detail can bring effectiveness in work, impacting the quality of results.

- Creative muscles are activated through meditation. A person practicing meditation will be better placed to generate creative ideas. Inventors, writers and original thinkers use meditation in some way to discover new grounds.

- Swift Meditation is the starting step to reach the

higher levels of meditation. It removes the fear and complexity associated with the practice of meditation.

- Meditation directly impacts the relations with other human beings which is important for social life and business. You can manage your bad emotions in a better way while strengthening positive emotions.

- Meditation is the reason for the most important connection, with self. It means that you are happy with yourself, the way you are, or the actions you take. This is important for confidence, self-belief and self-esteem.

People Using the Power of Meditation

There is no restriction to Swift Meditation based on age, race, region, language, religion or educational qualifications. It can be used by any human being due to its simplicity and impact. The meaning of Swift Meditation is the meditation that can be achieved simply and instantaneously. Once the initial state of meditation is achieved then it is the choice of the individual to go deeper. People unable to use meditation even after years of effort find Swift Meditation as an easy tool to achieve the state of meditation.

- It can be used by schoolchildren to deal with the anxiety of exams or to face the new environment of the school. Swift Meditation helps them in improving the aptitude and comprehension in studies.

- Swift Meditation is beneficial for public speakers, for example, just before an important speech or presentation. On stage, a speaker may feel a high level of anxiety or fear, disturbing normal breathing patterns. Swift Meditation can help in bringing the breathing to normal levels.

- It can be used by professionals to bring instant clarity to their minds. Executives are bombarded with unmanageable tasks and information, which seems difficult to manage. Swift Meditation can bring necessary clarity about the decisions to be taken based on available information for value maximization.

- Stress has become a normal part of life, even for kids. It has always been difficult to teach kids to meditate, as they lack patience and have difficulty in concentration. They can use Swift Meditation to start their journey towards meditation and use it to develop themselves mentally and physically.

- Older people may feel depressed due to their challenges and problems due to age or finances. They have lesser control over their life events due to their deteriorating physical health. Swift Meditation can help them energize their day to bring happiness and peace of mind for themselves and others.

- Other professionals working in high-stress conditions and situations like police officers, military personals, oil rigs professionals, fire workers and other people working in challenging environments, can use Swift Meditation to relax. These professionals do not have enough time or space to practice meditation, but they can use Swift Meditation to manage their stress in few minutes.

This is not Swift Meditation

- It is not a magic pill to solve all your problems,

instead, it will make you more efficient to face the challenges more effectively.

- Swift Meditation is not intended for deeper meditation, which is the advanced level of meditation. It is not the replacement of meditation, instead its starting process.

- It is also not the replacement of the physical activity and exercises required for physical fitness. Meditation is an integral part of yoga or any other physical activity focused on the improvement of the body.

- Swift Meditation is not a shortcut for anything. To develop any skill or competency, required time and defined efforts will be required. Swift Meditation can only make you a better learner with a relaxed mind.

- Swift Meditation removes the negativity from the mind to allow performance at a peak level. It will help you to think better, act efficiently and perform effectively.

The Meaning of Meditation

How many people know the true meaning of meditation?

Even with meditation becoming the buzzword of the present time, most people do not understand the true meaning of meditation. It is falsely considered as a religious practice or an ancient activity related to saints or synonymous with yoga. Meditation can be considered as a mental yoga or exercise to free the mind from thoughts, allowing it to relax deeply. A refreshed mind is ready to think and act with renewed energy to perform excellently. This is what everyone desires.

The Life Before Meditation

Whenever we think about meditation one common image

pops up in the mind, a person sitting on the floor with closed eyes. This person looks like a saint or a spiritual being, somehow getting connected to God. This image itself is confusing and disconnected from a normal person. Only a few people can visualize themselves resembling the image of meditation they have in their minds.

This is one of the biggest misconceptions about meditation. They only visualize the physical form but ignore the mental elements involved in the process. Many books, blogs, videos and the presence of complicated material make the whole process even more complex. It seems that meditation is reserved for some special people, which requires sacrifice and punishing schedule. This thinking has kept most people away from the blessings of meditation.

The objective of Swift Meditation is to introduce the process of meditation to the world with no complexity. People can experience the benefits and the power of meditation immediately, without years of practice or sacrifice.

Even now any human mind is full of thoughts that are generated either consciously or subconsciously. The five senses of the body are constantly busy capturing information from the environment and pushing it to the brain for analysis.

Every event or action, both real or virtual, is producing innumerable thoughts. For example, a bright red color car with a unique concept shape can raise several thoughts in the mind and a pungent smell can raise numerous questions. Similarly, a sudden temperature change can make anyone uncomfortable, forcing the mind to search for the reasons, while the sound of a siren can raise the threat level of mind, making it alert. These senses are constantly responding to the stimulus from their surroundings, filling the mind with an unending stream of thoughts.

Even if you minimize the number of senses by closing eyes and sitting comfortably in a calm place, without getting disturbed by anyone, the stream of thoughts will not stop. The mind will construct images that can be viewed even with closed eyes and virtual sound could be created for ears. Similarly, the mind will generate thoughts from the past or create new ones to fill the mind with an interminable stream of thoughts. You will be surprised to see the power of the mind to keep you engaged. Most of these thoughts will be vague, with no meaning, many will be negative while only a few will be positive. Even after the best efforts, it is difficult to stop this torrent of thoughts. Even if you free your mind for few seconds, the thoughts will be back again in full force. This is true for most of humanity.

The Process of Meditation

Meditation simply makes the mind hollow, free of thoughts. This is the only requirement for meditation. All the ideas and methodologies present in the world aim at driving out the thoughts from the mind, which is extremely difficult. The flow of thoughts always keeps the mind jam-packed. This doesn't allow you to think deeply or creatively. Only a minority of people in the world can think deeply. Stress is also the product of irrelevant thoughts. The mind working at full capacity on senseless thoughts can only produce minimal productive output. It can be considered like an efficient machine that can either be used effectively to create value or its energy is wasted in noise.

The process of meditation will aim to bring your focus to a specific act, so that focus from unrelated thoughts is slowly shifted, reducing the flow of thoughts in mind. It is also important that our senses minimize capturing information from the environment to flood the mind for processing. Therefore, it is necessary to choose the right place to meditate where most of our senses lie dormant, without the presence of any stimulus. It is also suggested to close your eyes before starting the process of meditation, as visual senses capture the maximum amount of information from the environment. The seasoned practitioners of meditation can meditate even with open eyes, as they can detach the information captured by the eye from the mind.

The methodology to focus can be varied, depending on the choice of the person and its suitability. Maybe a specific method is effective for a person which could differ completely from another. Some ways to focus could be:

- <u>Focus on breathing</u>– In this process a practitioner would focus on the details of breathing, the way a person is inhaling or exhaling. As the focus on breathing deepens, the flow of thoughts reduces.

- <u>Focus on music</u>– Instrumental music can be an effective way to meditate. Most of the modern mediation is based on music. In this process, the focus is diverted from thoughts to slow and calm instrumental music played at low volume. This is also used to relax the mind of people struggling with stress. Music is useful to deepen sleep as a relaxed mind experiences better sleep.

- <u>Focus on a humming sound produced by mouth</u>– This is similar to the previous point, only the music is replaced by a humming sound produced by mouth. Generally, it is the sound of Oohmm, in which the sound of 'm' is stretched long till the whole breath is consumed. Then a deep breath is taken and the process starts again while breathing out.

- <u>Visualization</u>– This method of meditation uses the power of mental visualization to create images, real or imaginary. These images can either be real, events that have occurred, or fictitious, which are created purely by the mind. This is a simple way to meditate and does not completely free us from thoughts. The main purpose of meditation using this method is to take control of the subconscious mind and shift it to the conscious mind, which is creating imaginary images.

- <u>Focus on a physical Act</u>– In this way, the meditative state is achieved by focusing on a specific physical activity. Breathing is an automatic physical act that has been discussed before. This process is different as the physical act is conscious, not automatic. It means that a physical act is performed consciously and repeatedly to drive the focus of the mind on the details of the act. For example, a simple slow tap on the table with an index finger can be a physical act done consciously. We can drive our complete attention to the action, which can help in freeing the mind with thoughts. Similarly, simple acts can be identified based on choice.

Part-Meditations

People have experienced meditation while doing something they love and feel connected with. They get completely engrossed in the work they are doing while getting disconnected from the outer world. For example, a person playing a musical instrument like a piano can get engrossed while playing the music, which can be considered as a part-meditation. it is not pure meditation but can give similar focus and relaxation and freedom from thoughts. Similarly, a person engaged in her work will feel meditative as she loves doing it. A singer can get into a meditative state while singing a beautiful song. This state is called the 'State of Flow', when a person feels floating in work, without experiencing the passage of time. People of faith can feel part-meditation while praying to God. The strong feeling of connection, with someone or something, can be meditative.

Those who are unable to concentrate with closed eyes can experience part-meditation while focusing their attention on an object or the image of a point. The process of part-meditation is by staring at the object or the image consistently with the purpose to drive the whole attention of mind towards the target. With constant practice, part-meditation can be experienced by managing all the senses and reducing the number of thoughts. This could be the first step towards meditation.

A large percentage of the world's population must have experienced the state of part-meditation in some form while doing something or being someone they love. Meditation is natural to the human mind. A healthy mind would require a meditative state for some time every day. It is difficult to maintain a dedicated schedule of meditation with a busy lifestyle. As most of humanity is trapped in unending work, people search for alternative ways to concentrate and relax. They may go for a walk in the jungle, tracking on the hills and engaging themselves in their hobbies. Some confused individuals would even use intoxicating substances like cigarettes, alcohol or drugs to disconnect themselves from reality, damaging their body and mind.

It is essential to have clarity about meditation with the right and effective ways to experience it.

Meditation is Natural

Meditation is natural to humans. The capacity of the human brain is still unknown to the scientific community. It is mysteriously strong and deep. Meditation can help in unlocking the secrets of the mind for effective usage. People who regularly meditate have better control over their emotions, make better decisions and are more creative. They are sharp learners and have an optimistic attitude with better perspectives about everything.

The human mind thrives in a state of calm and mental peace. Meditation ensures the state of deep relaxation, even deeper than sleep. A relaxed mind is more efficient, creative and is ready to solve problems. A tranquil mind can take clear decisions with confidence to get results.

Over several millenniums, the challenges faced by humans

changed every century, but the source of solution remained the same, a strong mind. In present times, the challenges for survival have reduced but were replaced by other complexities of life and work. Meditation has been at the forefront to deal with anxiety and stress. Yoga and meditation have become the buzzword of social media and Google search. People are looking for genuine solutions of ancient times, instead of superficial packages available for a price, which at most provide feel-good feeling, temporarily.

The discovery of meditation is similar to the discovery of fire, it was always present, only ready to be discovered. Still, the depths of meditation are yet to be revealed, unlocking the secrets of the mind. The present knowledge of meditation is enough to make the life of every human better. The objective of Swift Meditation is to let everyone take the benefits of meditation by making the process simple and Swift.

Life with Meditation

Once the meditation is experienced, regularly practiced and integrated into daily life, transformation happens. The mood swings vanish while positive emotions take the front seat.

Negative emotions are better managed and actions become effective with clear decision-making.

One of the most important elements of meditation is the enhancement of EQ – emotional quotient. The control over emotions makes them our strength, not weakness. If emotions can be understood and managed effectively, that would affect our life and performance directly. Meditation tends to strengthen our positive emotions and allow us to control our negative emotions effectively. This newfound power will enable us to deal with personal and professional challenges in a mature way.

Meditation is extremely effective to deal with stress. Regular practice of meditation will not let stress build-up. People have started to adopt meditative practices to deal with problems associated with stress. Meditation is now a buzzword in the corporate world. It is commonly used with discussions about spirituality, even without understanding its true meaning. To understand meditation, it must be experienced.

People can have different experiences with meditation. For some, it could be the control over emotions, for others it could be the clarity of mind, while some would discover health benefits with meditation. Following enhancements in life could be experienced once meditation becomes a part of life.

- For most people meditation is synonymous with relaxation. It helps in dealing with the daily stress that can build up due to personal or professional reasons. This directly affects the performance in work and improving the quality of life. Meditation is now considered one of the best stress management tools.

- The regular practice of meditation is an effective way to use emotions for adding value to your life. Human feelings are natural to every person but for most people emotions control their life. Meditation allows a person to have more control over their strong emotions helping them to think and act better.

- Meditation can be the path towards a calm mind. As the flow of thoughts is effectively managed, the mind can experience less noise, making it efficient. Mind without confusion is also better for taking decisions and living a good life.

- A meditative mind is also a creative mind. Creative people use meditation as a way to generate new ideas or develop new solutions. Without irrelevant thoughts, the mind's energy can be focused in a more productive way to create something new.

- Motivation and enthusiasm to solve problems are related to self-confidence, knowledge and experience. A clear and focused mind can excel in solving problems using microanalysis and troubleshooting. Meditation directly affects the performance and productivity of a person, a team or the whole organization.

- The growth in life can be ensured only with a constant stream of challenges. A person ignoring or avoiding challenges will be unable to find opportunities to learn and grow. A business expands revenues, market share and profitability if leaders are ready to challenge themselves to develop innovative quality products at optimal cost. A similar concept is relevant for any professional career. Meditation will be the constant source of clarity and energy for taking challenges and getting results.

- There is no doubt that a life with meditation is a life with fulfillment and peace of mind, which are the fundamental living objectives of every intelligent being.

- Most of the spiritual practices are associated with meditation in some form. Almost all religions use the concept of meditation in different formats to connect with their Gods. Even people who want to connect with themselves, meditation is the right way.

People can have different reasons to use meditation or discover new benefits further in their lives, but it always adds value in some way or the other. People are now discovering new uses and benefits of meditation to enhance their lives. Meditation has always been with human beings and will always remain a powerful tool to manage their mind.

Sitting Ideal vs Sitting in Meditation

To understand the concept of meditation in a different way let's do a small exercise. Right now, if you can manage the next 10 minutes without disturbance, then sit down doing nothing for 10 minutes. You can read forward after completing this exercise.

Let's introspect.

- Did you do it for 10 minutes or less?

- How was the experience?

- How do you feel?

- Could you complete it without any problem?

- What all came to your mind?

- How active were your five senses?

- How did you feel about the passing of time?

- Can you do it better next time?

After completing this exercise and answering these questions you must have understood the challenge in sitting ideal, without any thoughts in mind or doing anything. Now, if I extend the same exercise for two hours, I am sure that most people would raise objections about the time duration, as a couple of hours of meditation without practice would be torturous. Even if you complete that exercise, you will dread doing it again. You will notice that even if you were sitting ideal, your mind was not at rest. It was working hard to keep you busy even with weird thoughts, actions and activities. This experience would be tiring and unpleasant.

Is this experiment some form of meditation? No, it is not.

Meditation is the exact opposite of this experience. From a distance, visually both may look similar but are opposite. Look closer and the difference will be evident. A person in meditation will be calm, joyful and in control. Meditation is a process of relaxing your mind and body, making you energetic and in control. The process of meditation is not repulsive, instead, practitioners keep increasing the practice duration as the experience is incredibly fulfilling. The senior practitioners can sit in the state of meditation for hours, daily. Top business professionals and political leaders have found value in it and have made it a part of their daily life. People become more creative, focused and active even after meditating for few minutes every day. Meditation makes the life of a person better and most make it a daily habit or a ritual to meditate for some time.

Once the concept of Swift Meditation is learned it can be practiced to experience the difference between sitting ideal and in meditation.

Meditation Data

In the last few decades, meditation has been adopted exponentially all over the world. It is estimated that around 200 to 500 million people meditate in some form worldwide. According to a report from the 'Center for Disease Control and Prevention', in the year 2020, over 16% of Americans meditated at least once in the last 12 months. This is a notable appreciation since 2012 when only 4% of Americans had meditated the previous year. The major reasons for this increase include mobile apps for meditation and yoga, stressful conditions due to COVID-19, acceptance of meditation by corporations and integration of meditation classes at schools and colleges. Few other sources have confirmed this number could be higher, up to 40%, if religious meditative practices of different groups are included.

General wellness is the primary motive for 76% of the people using meditation, while 60% use it for boosting their energy levels and 50% use it for improving memory, focus and relieving anxiety, stress and depression. 65% of practitioners reported about 60% reduction in their anxiety levels after nine months of meditation. As meditation reduces anxiety and stress levels, it can reduce the risk of being hospitalized for heart diseases by 85%. In 75% of insomnia cases meditation helped, while 90% of insomniacs reduced or eliminated the use of medication. 57% of women practicing meditation noticed the reaction in physical and psychological PMS symptoms.

Meditation has physical benefits too. The regular practice improved the ability of practitioners with back pain by 30%. The PTSD (post-traumatic stress disorder) symptoms were reduced in 73% of the cases, though further research is yet to be done. 80% of the practitioners lowered their blood pressure and could use lesser medication to manage it, while 16% stopped taking medicine for hypertension. The practice of meditation is also good for memory and improving the attention span within a week. According to a Harvard study, the daily practice of meditation can increase grey matter in the hippocampus.

According to a US-based health survey, more women (16.3%) used meditation compared to men (11.8%). More white adults (15.2%) used meditation compared to Blacks (13.5%) and Hispanics (10.9%). People in the age group of 45 to 64 are most likely (16%) to use meditation compared to other age brackets, which are always 3 to 4 percent less.

According to religious groups, 66% of United States Buddhists, 49% of evangelical Protestants, 77% of Jehovah's Witnesses and 25% of atheists meditate at least once a week. Percentage of children using meditation increased 10 times (to 6%) since 2012 (0.6%). More teenagers (7%) use meditation compared to other children groups (5%).

More than half of Fortune 1000 companies provided a mindfulness class to their employees in the year 2019, which is an appreciable increase from 36% in the year 2017. Why? A limited study found that meditation has the potential to increase employees' productivity by 120%, decrease absenteeism by 85% and increase profits by 520%. This explains the fact about the increasing number of schools introducing meditation to their students.

In the year 2021, Meditation Market is expected to cross the size of USD 2 billion, which will grow consistently in the next decade. The meditation Market will account for revenues of USD 9.0 billion by 2027 growing at a CAGR of 10.40%.

The growth in the users of meditation shows it is receiving acceptability in different regions and cultures of the world. People are looking for alternative ways to manage their mental health, other than psychological medications.

Top mobile applications in 2020 for meditation are Calm, Headspace, Meditopia, Yoga Go, Breethe and Meditation App. These apps have millions of subscriptions.

Science Backed Benefits of Meditation

Productivity and Performance Benefits

1. Improves multitasking: as meditation improves focus, it is beneficial for the professionals dealing with multitasking.

2. Improves memory: comprehension and retention enhance drastically after a month of the regular practice of meditation.

3. Enhances attention span: meditation is found to strengthen the area of the brain associated with attentiveness.

4. Boosts creativity: meditation is found useful in both enhancing creativity and searching for solutions.

5. Analytical skills: meditation can make a person a better thinker with problem-solving skills.

6. Deeper sleep: the relaxation achieved with meditation

can help to sleep better.

Health Benefits

1. Reduce inflammation: inflammation caused due to stress and anxiety can be managed and reduced.
2. Minimizes pain: regular practitioners of meditation have reported ease at managing pain.
3. Boosts immune system: it has been scientifically proven that meditation enhances the community against the virus and bacteria.
4. Lowers blood pressure: this is one of the most commonly reported advantages of meditation, which is directly related to anxiety and stress.
5. Reduces cortisol levels: blood cortisol levels were observed to be reduced by 20% after a week of meditation.
6. Lowers oxygen consumption: meditation can relax the body and mind even deeper than sleep, reducing the consumption of oxygen by 20%.

Improved Social Life

1. Compassion: meditation makes a person more compassionate and caring for other humans and

animals.

2. Emotions management: it has been proven scientifically that the practice of meditation can enhance the part of the brain that promotes regulation of emotions and response control.

3. Social connectedness: meditation can make you more aware of your surroundings and the emotions of other people. It will improve your connection with other people, even strangers.

4. Relationships: a calm mind and control over words are necessary to build and maintain relations. Meditation can help in developing this skill.

5. Anxiety management: meditation can help in the management of anxiety and fear, which are responsible for speech disorders and panic attacks.

A Small Percentage of People Use Meditation

For long it seemed like a fad, just like any business hot topic with a short life. But now people are acknowledging the benefits of meditation and accepting its value. It is now extensively being used for social and business environments.

Educational institutes regularly organize training programs to introduce meditation to students. Most people who have experienced it have endorsed its positive impact.

Till the start of the 21ˢᵗ century, the practice of meditation was restricted due to the limited availability of training centers. Now, the meditation training is easily accessible, in online and physical formats. This is slowly gaining the status of a lifestyle practice. People love to use it for health benefits and for healing themselves. Meditation enhances the value of other practices like yoga and martial art. No one has ever found any negative in the practice of meditation. It has no negative side effects.

Meditation can easily be confused with any spiritual practice. Though it can be the starting point of many special processes, it is much more than a spiritual connection. Many orthodox religious groups or uninformed people consider the practice of meditation associated with a specific religious practice, instead, it is a holistic way to control and manage psychological systems. It is natural to the human body and mind. Meditation can transform the life of a person, making it better.

The practice of meditation can look complex and formidable,

not accessible to normal humans. But, as more people understand and utilize the concept of meditation, it is becoming a common part of a high percentage of educated individuals. The majority now understands that meditation is not much different from any physical exercise which requires certain motivation and time management to integrate into the daily schedule of life. It may also seem tough to practice as the person absorbed in meditation may look forced and strained, instead, it is the opposite. The time of meditation is most relaxed and joyful.

The practice of meditation may look dissimilar from the modern way of living. The present generation has always lived with the latest gadgets, connectivity, innumerable choices and instant gratification. A conscious choice, consistency and discipline are necessary to introduce meditation in the lifestyle, as it requires the position and state dissimilar from their normal activities. Once the practitioners experience the state of meditation, they understand its value and reason. Meditation cannot be forced. It is always the choice of the individuals to make it a part of their life.

Marketing and advertising are the major influence to persuade people to buy and consume. A product or service is repackaged by marketing professionals to make it look cool and trendy. The teachers and trainers of meditation rarely believe in advertising packages to attract people. Most of the gym-based exercise routines and equipment are flashing, fancy dressed and are presented as a Hollywood movie. That is the reason cardio exercises routines looks much cooler than meditation or yoga. it is believed that meditation does not need marketing muscles or advertising brains to sell its value preposition to interested people. The adaptation of meditation depends only upon the need, choice and experience.

It is believed by many unaware groups about the necessity of training is only for the body, not the mind. The same ignorant belief holds for healing after an accident, trauma or disease. The truth is that the mind can heal itself slowly with time, without any external help or attention. But the right actions can help it rebuild itself much stronger, faster and better. The mind's capacity is much more than normally understood and used by people. Meditation can help in unlocking it.

The Inaccessibility of Meditation

The fundamental reasons are understanding and experience.

Most people do not understand the true concept of meditation and consider it something else, which does not allow them to explore it further. Another reason is the lack of experience of the transformative powers of meditation, which can improve them mentally and physically. Momentary pause from daily life to sit with yourself is the only requirement to understand and experience meditation.

Cannot Experience Meditation

Meditation benefits cannot be achieved with faulty understanding and wrong execution. Many fake experts have created their own (mostly wrong) versions of meditation. They market it heavily to make it profitable like a successful fresh startup. Their propaganda is responsible to confuse normal people about the implementation of the genuine meditation principle.

In the world of people practicing meditation rarely do people complain. Ironically, it is not difficult to find people who have not experienced the advantages of meditation even after practicing for some time. According to them, they doing everything right but are unable to discover any benefits of their efforts.

What wrong are they doing?

The practice of meditation is not a recent concept instead existed since humans found consciousness. It was practiced for thousands of years in different forms, used all over the world. It could be that people unable to experience meditation needs correction or some modifications in their practice.

Following is a list of common mistakes people make, restricting their experience with meditation.

- Even though the concept of meditation is not complex, it requires understanding the concept before experiencing it. It is wrong to rush through it. There is no shortcut to meditation. This experience must be earned through understanding it deeply and practicing with discipline.

- Meditation cannot be experienced by doing it casually. Without belief, it is difficult to bring sincerity into any endeavor. If this practice is taken as a game or a tourist visit, then it is difficult to experience its power. A belief can be developed only with genuine interest and investing time to understand the practice of meditation. Many people are unable to commit the required amount of time and energy to earn the benefits of mediation.

- Attitude defines the behavior of a person. Without the right attitude, appropriate actions cannot be taken for desired results. Actions also depend upon the need to do something. As people do not understand the concept of meditation, they seldom understand its power. It may take a certain time and sincere practice until they experience meditation. The lack of knowledge does not allow them to put genuine efforts into meditation.

- Lack of patience is the biggest cause that people are unable to experience meditation. To get expertise and required deepness in meditation may require time, discipline and regularity, without which the advantages of meditation cannot be experienced.

- A small percentage of people do not want to experience meditation as they do it only to find shortcomings. They are fault finders and they can criticize anything and everything. As they don't want, they cannot experience meditation.

The Practice of Swift Meditation

The following section specifies several techniques to practice and experience Swift Meditation. Each segment discusses the fundamental idea, the logic of using the technique and the way to practice it. Remember to keep your comfort level as the indicator to inform about the level of intensity each exercise is to be practiced. These exercises can be slightly modified based on your requirements and needs. One or more of the following techniques can be used to get into Swift Meditation state. If one idea is working for you well then you don't need to use others, though it is good to experience other methods too.

First Technique: T1– 10-10

Summary: 10-second breathing pause, 10 deep focused breaths

10-10: The Idea

This idea uses breathing as the focus area for Swift Meditation. This technique is based on creating the conditions to compel the mind to lose attention to irrelevant thoughts and diverting the complete attention to breathing. The best way to force the mind to focus on breathing is by pausing it momentarily. As breathing is essential for living, the momentary pause will activate the threat segment of the mind to restart the breathing. This will be an instantaneous process. As the mind will search for the reasons for breathing interruptions, the thoughts in the mind will have degraded priority, allowing the mind to lose focus on the stream of thoughts coming to the mind. That is the moment for the mind to feel relaxed and get ready to absorb energy to perform better.

10-10: The Action

This technique uses a higher priority activity to divert attention from irrelevant thoughts to something that matters. The mind is engaged in several unconscious activities like breathing, which are essential for the living body. Any disruption in these activities will trigger the threat segment of the mind to take immediate action. This process will be instant as the survival mechanism will have higher priority than the vague thoughts in mind. This process will drive out unnecessary thoughts from the mind to look for the reasons for interruptions and to take immediate action to restore normal breathing.

10-10: The Reasons

The top priority of the survival mechanism is the automatic action of the mind to surpass any activity to attend to the emergency at hand. The mind would focus on any activity disturbing its normal functioning for correction. That is the normal way to ensure that body keeps working properly. As all necessary precautions are taken, the real risk is minimized but the natural focus on the exercise would reduce the number of thoughts in mind to minimal. This can help in achieving Swift Meditation.

10-10: The Process

The step-by-step process of implementing the technique of 10-10 to experience Swift Meditation is as follows.

The process for the exercise is:

- Sit in a comfortable position where you will not be disturbed during the process of the Swift Meditation exercise. Though the process of experiencing Swift Meditation works even in the standing position but sitting position is better as it has less strain on muscles. Even the lying position can also be used in this exercise but it may put the practitioner to sleep (due to relaxation), which you may not want at that moment.

- The next step is to reduce the number of stimulations for active senses. This can be achieved by sitting in a quiet place free of odors and surprises. Closing the eyes would reduce the number of visible stimuli and keeping the mouth free of any eatables would help in Swift Meditation.

- For the next 20 seconds try to consciously drive the thoughts out of your mind as much as possible. Do this by focusing the attention on the count of 1 to 20 as you whisper them with the gap of 1 second between two numbers.

- Now, start the process of 10 – 10. In this process hold the breath for 10 seconds then take 10 deep breaths. Repeat this process 10 times. Use nose to breath-in and mouth to breath-out.

- It is important that while deep breaths are taken, the focus must be completely on the breaths as we inhale and exhale.

- This process of Swift Meditation is a good relaxation technique that will help in gaining better control over emotions.

10-10: Points to take care

The more you practice the better the command over the Swift Meditation process.

10-10: Precautions to be taken

It's important to feel comfortable all the time while practicing Swift Meditation. If you feel uncomfortable, discontinue the exercise.

Second Technique: T2– Flashback

Summary: Take any event in the last 24 hours and see it again in mind with details.

Flashback: The Idea

This idea uses the power of visualization and focuses to drive out the irrelevant thoughts from the mind to concentrate on something consciously. The events of the past few hours are fresh in our minds, saved with minute details, even if not consciously observed. These details are captured and saved in our subconscious mind, which can be extracted with conscious focus. This technique will use the said ability of the mind to focus by extracting the details of the chosen event. This involves the ability of the mind to visualize and concentrate to search for the details and express them through words. It is like watching a video film in your mind of a past event in color and at the desired speed. While working on this exercise we are unaware that this technique has helped us to drive out most of the thoughts of our mind and helped us to part meditate.

Flashback: The Action

The purpose of the technique is to divert the attention of the conscious mind to the immediate past activities fresh in our mind. As the conscious mind concentrates to focus attention on the event (please make sure that a positive and pleasant event is chosen), the mind gets freed from the unrelated thoughts present in the mind. It also helps in interrupting the constant stream of thoughts constantly engaging the mind. Indeed, the mind will not be completely free of all the thoughts but the technique has minimized it and has focused the attention on some specific thoughts which are neither tiring nor negative. The mind is powerful enough to manage effectively a set a few thoughts while freeing the rest of the brain to help it relax.

Flashback: The Reason

The technique is simple enough to be used by most to

practice Swift Meditation. The events of the last few hours are generally fresh in mind, which can be remembered in minute details if required. Visualization is a powerful way to focus on something, which can even direct attention from most other areas. The technique involves watching an immediate event that is effortless and interesting. This is an effective process that can help in experiencing Swift Meditation.

Flashback: The Process

Before starting we need to identify an event to be visualized. This incident can be of past few hours still fresh in mind which can be remembered in minute details.

- Before starting the process of meditation, identify a place where you can sit for some time without disturbance. We also need to identify a comfortable place to practice where none of your senses is stimulated either through rapid movements, loud noise, strong odor or anything else which can disturb you while visualizing. This is necessary to experience Swift Meditation with no disturbance.

- Eyes should be closed during the process of meditation to block the sense of sight, which is the prime sense of thought generation.

- Visualize the chosen event in your mind. This process will be similar to watching a video file on a television screen in which the event is being played. The event will be viewed in slow motion to make you focus on every detail of the video. For example, the video of the event will be played at one-fourth of the speed to ensure capturing every detail like the color of the clothes, name of the book, an odd object kept in the corner or other details not normally observed consciously. This activity requires deep focus for observation, allowing the mind to get freedom from the stream of thoughts in mind.

- We may move forward or backward at the desired speed, just like in a video player. This will allow us to focus on the scenes in which most of the data is stored in the subconscious mind.

- With regular practice, deeper meditation can be achieved through this process.

- The time duration of meditation is the choice of the practitioner but five minutes of practice in one session should be minimum.

- This process can be used at any time of the day and as and when required. For regular practice, we suggest that practice for 5-10 minutes, two times every day.

Flashback: Points to take care

- Choose only good, positive and pleasant events for visualization.

- Keep the stimulants for your five senses away or minimal to reduce the instances of disturbances.

- Keep the video visualization slow to focus on each frame of the event.

Flashback: Precautions

- Use no bad or negative event for visualization.

- Do not use the Swift Meditation process for a long time as that could be disorienting. Our objective is to gain freedom the thoughts and relax not to detach ourselves from reality.

Third Technique: T3– World Not Seen Before

Summary: Flashback technique to see the world not seen before.

World Not Seen Before: The Idea

This technique is the extension of the previous "Flashback" technique, in which we visualized an immediate previous event in our mind. In this process, we will go into the details of each scene by zooming in. For example, in a scene of a garden, the green benches kept at the corner can be zoomed-in to check the details of the material, texture and color fading due to exposer. Next, a plant can be zoomed-in to check the color and size of the leaves and flowers. Similarly, different areas can be identified to zoom-in to check the details of the images in our minds. This visualization should be vivid to stimulate the five senses with visuals, smell, sound, taste and touch. The experience is soothing and satisfactory.

World Not Seen Before: The Action

This technique uses the process of visualization to create images in our minds and checking the minute details. Visualization is a powerful technique to focus our attention on a specific event playing in our minds. It will free our mind from unrelated thoughts, instantly with little effort. A free mind can automatically learn the process to speed up the process of meditation. The mind is a master player in visualization and creating stuff, it can even find or fill in details not even present in the real event. It is like creating a story both with real and fictional elements.

World Not Seen Before: The Reason

The process of visualization is an intense technique to capture the energy and focus of the mind. Zooming in and checking the minute details of images in mind will be a step forward to utilize the resources of visualization to achieve deeper focus. This could be the starting point in your journey to deeper meditation.

World Not Seen Before: The Process

To use this process of Swift Meditation slowly observe the things around you with the objective of consciously capture the minute details from the scene. Take as much time as required to be comfortable.

- Before starting the process of meditation, identify a place to practice for some time without disturbance. You also need to identify a comfortable place to sit where none of your senses is stimulated either through rapid movements, loud noise, strong odor or anything that can disturb during meditation. This is necessary to experience Swift Meditation with no disturbance.

- Eyes should be closed during the process of meditation to block the sense of sight, which is the prime sense of thought generation.

- Think about an event of immediate past fresh in the memory. Close your eyes to re-live that moment again. It is like going to the past virtually, in your mind. The objective is to visualize deep to get to the details of the objects and things, even the minute specifications. Try to capture the little specifics like color, unique design, geometric patterns, fabric or texture. In this exercise we are not interested in the emotional aspect of the event, only the visual perspective must be considered.

- If you do not remember any details then allow the mind to create them and fill the gaps through visualization.

- As your mind is focused on capturing the details of the event with closed eyes, the mind will be free from the thoughts without any relevance.

World Not Seen Before: Points to take care

- Remember this process is for relaxation, not to strain your mind or body. If you are feeling any stress then it indicates a need for correction.

- If you feel uncomfortable in any way, stop the

exercise.

World Not Seen Before: Precautions

- Visualize no negative or painful thoughts, focus only on the positive.

- You can put an alarm to come out of your meditation process after a certain time. Choose the time duration most comfortable for you. With regular practice, the time duration can be increased.

Fourth Technique: T4– Stretched Focus

Summary: Finding focus in a stretched yoga position

Stretched Focus: The Idea

Yoga is a well-known set of stretching exercises for improving overall health. Yoga and meditation go hand in hand to enhance mental and physical wellbeing. Practicing meditation with yoga is natural and easy to learn. A set of muscles is stretched in a position (asana) of yoga and mental focus is concentrated on that stretched muscle. We can feel the slow contraction and expansion of the muscle and the flow of blood through it. We can even feel the warmth and the heat produced due to muscle stretching. During yoga, several vibrant activities are transpiring simultaneously in the body, which is enough to drive out most thoughts from the mind. The mind freed from thoughts can experience meditation, instantly.

Stretched Focus: The Action

This technique is employing the energetic practice of yoga to sit in a stretched muscle position to free the mind from irrelevant thoughts and experience Swift Meditation. Yoga is relaxing for the body helping the mind to meditate by creating conditions to focus the attention of the mind on a specific activity. People have used this technique for thousands of years to achieve deeper meditation. We will use this technique for Swift Meditation.

Stretched Focus: The Reason

The brain is the most powerful organ of any living body. Mind resides in the physical brain. The mind is full of energy to make it dynamic and active. An idle mind is also busy with hundreds of irrelevant thoughts running through the mind to grab your attention. Even a person busy in an activity will have a large portion of the mind engaged in thoughts with no meaning. To free the mind from these tiring thoughts the mind must get engaged in any activity to capture its full attention and energy. Yoga, if performed correctly, can be an effective way to get into meditation. This process is also relaxing for the mind and body to make it a natural ally of meditation. With regular practice, yoga and meditation can be integrated easily.

Stretched Focus: The Process

Before using this technique, it is required to learn few yoga positions from master practitioners, either physically or through digital channels. These exercises must be performed in the right way, without mistakes to avoid any injury.

- To experience Swift Meditation through yoga, choose a simple yoga position in which a set of muscles is stretched. The muscle strain should be normal and not excessive. Our objective is to use the stretch in muscle to focus our mind on that specific muscle.

- Sit in a comfortable position, as required by yoga rules. Follow all the rules as specified by the trainers. We will hold the stretched yoga position for some time to experience Swift Meditation. Choose a nice place where most of your senses will not be stimulated through rapid motions, sound, odor or any other activity, which can disturb the focus and attention. Breathing should be normal and natural, slowly inhaling through the nose and exhaling through the mouth.

- The eyes should be closed to block the prime sense while getting into the yoga position (asana). Everything should be done slowly and we will be holding the stretched yoga position for some time to experience Swift Meditation.

- While keeping the eyes closed, focus attention on the stretched portion of the muscle. Visualize and experience the details of the contraction and expansion of the muscles and the flow of blood through the veins. Try to visualize and experience every activity happening in that specific muscle. Regular practice would allow us to do it better.

- This exercise can be repeated with different Yoga positions, focusing on different muscles.

Stretched Focus: Points to take care

- Remember to maintain a comfort level all the time,

both mentally and physically.

- Breathing must remain normal during the whole process of Swift Meditation.

Stretched Focus: Precautions

- This exercise needs to be performed with care as both mental and physical elements are engaged in it.

- Care needs to be taken to not overstretch the muscles involved in the exercise.

- Always remember to keep the synchronization of mental and physical faculties.

Fifth Technique: T5– That One Sense

Summary: Gaining mental focus with the activation of (only) one sense like touch on cold, beautiful music, eyes opened in dark, fresh smell, tasting something amazing.

That One Sense: The Idea

Human senses are powerful sensors to capture information from the outside world. Each of the five human sensory perceptions (vision, hearing, touch, spatial orientation, smell, and taste) focuses on a specific area to collect information to be processed by the mind. Most of the thoughts are generated by processing data from the human senses. All human senses work simultaneously to define the world around us. But if we could concentrate on one chosen sense to focus complete attention of the mind, then the data captured by other senses will fall in priority to reduce the number of thoughts generated in the mind. For example, we could focus on a soothing natural smell with eyes closed in a noiseless place. Creative ways can be identified to use the power of one specific sense to focus the attention of the mind.

That One Sense: The Action

This technique is utilizing the power of the "information capture mechanism" of human senses to capture the attention of the mind. Every human sense is constantly working to capture the information about the environment to help the mind understand it. In this process, we will reduce the number of active senses to capture minimal information while enhancing the sensory perception of one specific sense to capture its minute details. This will be a unique experience for the mind which will divert its complete attention to experience Swift Meditation. This experience would be enjoyable and relaxing as one specific human sense is appreciated and admired.

That One Sense: The Reason

It is natural for humans to capture information from their active senses. A large percentage of the brain is engaged to process this information. Freeing the mind from this processing would allow it to consciously focus on the chosen area. This can be achieved instantly as senses are sensitive to capture data and the mind is receptive to absorb the information. Relieving the mind from irrelevant thoughts to focus on a specific area would be simultaneous. This will allow the mind to experience Swift Mediation.

That One Sense: The Process

The fundamental objective of this exercise is to focus on a specific sense while minimizing the sensation of other senses. This goal can be achieved by stimulating the chosen sense with strong stimulants while minimizing the opportunity for other senses to capture any information. This process uses the 'Focus on Present' to dive into Swift Meditation.

Before starting the process of Swift Meditation, choose one human sense to specifically focus on and create an environment suitable for it. For example, if chosen sense is Sound then the place of practice should be noise-free. We need to close our eyes (as the sense of sight may interfere with our focus on sound) and sit in a comfortable position, without strain on body muscles.

The process of using different senses for meditation are as follows:

1. **Sense of Sound**– Sit with closed eyes in a noise-free place and listen to pleasant soft instrumental music to focus. Make sure that none of the other senses are stimulated. With eyes closed, focus on the beautiful music by feeling it and observing its details. You can focus on each instrument played and the way the mechanics is used in producing the sound. Most thoughts will disappear, leaving you with a calm and stressless mind. Listen to an instrument (like the piano) and visualize all the details in it. The way key is pressed and all the components working together to produce the fine sound. If you have proximity to nature then use this exercise by listening to the sounds of nature.

2. **Sense of Smell**– Repeat the above exercise by replacing the music (or sounds of nature) with a pleasant smell. The natural smell would be better than artificial, which are generally chemically produced.

3. **Sense of Taste**– Repeat the above exercise with something soothing and tasty (like a bar of chocolate) in your mouth. Experience and visualize the fine details associated with the taste. Absorbing yourself in the taste would let you achieve Swift Meditation. For example, it could be the chocolate flavor you like or anything else. Observe the way the mouth and body react to the taste. Notice minute details by giving enough time to each activity.

4. **Sense of Touch**– Repeat the said exercise with something smooth or with texture. It could be slightly hot or cold. For example, it could be performed with a piece of ice, which is being touched for a few seconds with each fingertip. This exercise can be taken to a higher level by using touch to experience different properties of various materials, like capturing the minute details of the shape and texture of a designer box.

5. **Sense of Sight**– This is the most difficult exercise as sight captures a lot of information every second. We need to identify an object on which the focus needs to be fixed by staring it consistently. This

exercise may require some time to master. For example, you can watch a clock to observe and capture its minute details. You can follow the seconds' needle slowly moving forward every second and the slow moment of the minutes' needle and the way both are synchronized. You can also visualize the whole mechanics playing behind the front face of the clock to move the whole system and to keep the correct time. The more you observe and visualize the better you would experience Swift Meditation.

That One Sense: Points to take care

Ensure that you remain comfortable while doing the exercises.

Sixth Technique: T6- Draw the Circle

Summary: Draw a big circle on a piece of paper using your finger.

Draw the Circle: The Idea

In this exercise, we will use the sense of touch to manage an activity for driving the focus while allowing the thoughts to leave the mind. The mind without thoughts will be relaxed to regain energy.

Draw the Circle: The Action

The focus on the one specific sense would reduce attention to other senses while amplifying the attention on the minute activities related to touch. The mind would be registering all those micro activities which are generally ignored in daily life.

As the mind is busy capturing a constant stream of information, it becomes less active in generating irrelevant thoughts without any meaning or objective.

People who are good at concentrating their attention on a specific activity have trained their minds to divert their energy from pointless thoughts generated by the mind.

Draw the Circle: The Reason

This technique is using one of the five powerful senses of human beings, touch. As most people do not completely understand their senses deeply, these exercises would help them connect with their senses at a deeper level. In this exercise, we will use the sense of touch to connect with it deeply. Most people do not know that the deep connection with their senses can help them manage their thoughts in the mind. When all the senses are working simultaneously then it is difficult to manage the burst of information captured by all the senses which struggle for the significance to be processed by the mind.

Draw the Circle: The Process

The idea is simple. A big circle is to be drawn slowly on an A4 size paper using a finger. The objective is not to draw the circle on paper using ink or any other marker/ pen but to use the activity to activate and prioritize the sense of touch. As the circle is drawn extremely slowly with 1 mm movement in one second, which is 1 cm in 10 seconds. The circle is to be dawn full to reach the starting point after traveling the whole circumference of the circle.

A comfortable, quiet and clean place would be effective for this exercise. The identification of the right place of the activity can ensure minimizing the capture of information by other senses from the environment.

The correct execution of the exercise would take around 4 to 5 minutes to complete one circle. This exercise can be completed in half the time by completing half the circle depending upon the requirements and time limitations.

Draw the Circle: Points to take care

- It is the focus on the sense of touch to capture every detail about it while minimizing the absorption of information by other senses.

- Take a plain sheet of blank paper without creases.

- Keep the movement of the finger extremely slow.

Draw the Circle: Precautions

Do the exercise only if you feel connected with the idea and can experience Swift Meditation with the process.

Other Effective Techniques

The next portion briefly describes some more effective techniques for experiencing Swift Meditation. These techniques can be used with similar ideas as described in the previous section. Use a calm and comfortable place for practicing. The place of practice should minimize the information capture for human senses. Finally, modify the technique based on your requirements and limitations. If anything makes the practice uncomfortable, discontinue it.

Seventh Technique: T7- Look Closely Closed

In this exercise, capture a view in twenty seconds, then close your eyes to recreate it in your mind with minute details. This process will allow you to get into Swift Meditation as the mind will be focused on capturing as much information as possible within twenty seconds and then re-creating it in the mind. These virtual images can be verified after opening your eyes again and checking it with the initial view. The objective is not to recreate exactly the view in your mind, instead, it is to divert the attention of the mind towards an engaging task so that the mind could become free of irrelevant thoughts. This exercise is also good for improving your observation skills.

Eighth Technique: T8– Stretch and Release

In this exercise, the focus will be directed towards a specific muscle, which will be contracted and released slowly. For example, if the right thigh muscle is slowly contracted for 30 seconds and then released in a similar time duration while we try to divert the attention of mind towards this act. Be careful about not over-stretching or over-contracting any muscle. Special attention should be taken to minimize the information capture by other senses of the human body. With regular practice, any muscle can be targeted to experience Swift Meditation.

Ninth Technique: T9– Very Slow Movement

In the process of yoga, the slow moment of the body is essential to achieve the benefits of exercise. The slow moment of any part of the body captures the attention of the mind, allowing it to free itself from unwanted thoughts. The mind should be focused on capturing every detail of the movement. For example, while sitting in a comfortable position and minimizing the capture of information from our senses we can slowly lift our hand perpendicular to the body and then slowly lifting it all the way up to bring it in the line of the body length. It must be done extremely slowly to complete the whole act in 60 seconds. In the next minute, the hand can be brought back slowly to its original position. This simple act can be an effective tool in experiencing Swift Meditation if performed in the right way.

Though, the philosophy of this process is simple but is extremely engaging for the mind to capture its attention. This exercise can help drive out thoughts to experience Swift Meditation.

The Start of the Journey

This is the end of the book but start of your journey of meditation. The simple techniques of the book would allow experiencing meditation instantaneously at any place or time. Swift Meditation is an effective technique to relax and to gain clarity in mind. It will free mind from irrelevant thoughts to help you focus by improving concentration. This can be achieved by anyone, even without any practice. The most important contribution of Swift Meditation is its ability to make anyone experience freedom and power without dedicating themselves to the hard practice of meditation. Practitioners, who want to take the practice forward to achieve deeper meditation, the path becomes simpler. It will also allow the practitioners of Swift Meditation to gain clarity about the type of meditation suitable for them, helping them to choose the right path.

We hope to have added value to your life by introducing Swift Meditation. Now, you have the power to utilize your conscious and subconscious mind effectively to improve your life and work.

Happy meditation.

Copyright

Cataloging-in-Publication Data
Names: Pathak, Nilam -author. Sharma, Anshuman -author.
Title: Swift Meditation- Power to All / by Nilam Pathak,
Anshuman Sharma.
Includes bibliographical references and index.
Identifiers:
ISBN: 9798720820442

About Authors

Nilam Pathak

Nilam is an experienced communications professional who is the author of six books published internationally. She has worked with top brands to improve employee productivity and Human Resource Systems. She believes in strengthening the weaker sections of the society through communication and personality development. She is a proud mother of two daughters and lives in North India.

Anshuman Sharma

Anshuman is an entrepreneur, investor, and author who has been instrumental in creating many successful companies. He has more than eighteen years of holistic and rich experience in Consulting, Managing, Marketing and Selling products & services. He has created Private Limited companies like Aegis Consulting, Nexeia Technologies, Equifone Solutions and Meetle Technologies. He is also involved in supporting the development of several other companies.